SIMPLE CHAIR

EXERCISES FOR SENIORS

OVER 60

Stay active and independent with 50 easy and accessible workouts to boost your strength and flexibility

By

Franco Richard

Disclaimers

The exercises and activities described in this book involve physical movement and potential risks. The reader should understand that participation in any exercise program carries a risk of physical injury. It is recommended to consult with a healthcare professional before starting any exercise program, particularly if you have any pre-existing medical conditions or physical limitations.

The author and publisher disclaim any liability or loss in connection with the exercises, instructions, and advice contained in this book. The reader assumes full responsibility for their own actions and safety while engaging in the exercises and activities described in this book.

Table of content

Thank you for choosing "Simple Chair Exercises for Seniors over 60" as your guide to staying active, independent, and boosting your strength and flexibility. I hope you will find this book informative and helpful in your fitness journey.

I would greatly appreciate it if you could take a moment to rate and review this book. Your feedback is valuable to me as it helps me improve and provide better content in the future. Your positive review will also encourage others to discover the benefits of chair exercises and lead a healthier lifestyle.

Your honest opinion is highly appreciated, and I thank you in advance for your support.

Stay active, stay independent, and keep moving!

Introduction

Keeping an independent and active lifestyle becomes more and more crucial as we get older. Not only does regular physical activity improve our general health, but it also enhances our quality of life. Maintaining an active lifestyle becomes crucial for seniors over 60 to maintain their independence and vitality.

Seniors can engage in safe and efficient workouts that improve strength, flexibility, and overall well-being by doing chair exercises. These exercises are accessible and appropriate for people with different levels of mobility or physical fitness because they are specifically made to be done from the comfort of a chair.

Seniors who perform chair exercises can gain a variety of advantages, such as:

1. Increased strength: Seniors can maintain and increase their strength with chair exercises, which focus on different muscle groups. Strength is essential for carrying out daily tasks with ease.

2. Improved flexibility: Regularly stretching and performing range-of-motion exercises while seated can help to increase flexibility, which will help to promote better joint mobility and lower the chance of injury.

3. Improved stability and balance: Balance exercises are a common part of chair workouts, and they can help seniors become more stable and less likely to fall.

4. Cardiovascular health: By raising heart rate and circulation, chair exercises can improve cardiovascular health even though they might not be as intense as conventional cardio workouts.

5. Mood and mental health: Research has demonstrated that physical activity, even when done while seated, releases endorphins, improves mood, and lessens the signs and symptoms of anxiety and depression.

I'll walk you through a number of simple chair exercises in this book that are geared especially for seniors over 60. With the help of these gentle yet efficient exercises, you can progressively increase your strength, flexibility, and general level of fitness. Warm-up, upper body, lower body, core, stretching, and cool-down exercises are among the various body regions that will be the focus of each chapter.

These chair exercises can be modified to fit your ability level, regardless of your current fitness level. There are numerous exercises that can be customized to meet your specific needs and fitness objectives, regardless of your level of experience.

The secret is to pay attention to your body, begin at a comfortable pace, and increase gradually as your confidence and ability grow.

You can actively support your own well-being, preserve your independence, and lead a full and active senior life by implementing these chair exercises into your daily routine. Together, let's take on this adventure and learn the delight of maintaining an active lifestyle while remaining independent with simple chair exercises.

Chapter 1

Warm-up exercises

We will look at a series of warm-up exercises in this chapter that will help your body prepare for the chair exercises that follow. Exercises for warming up the body are crucial for improving flexibility, blood flow, and muscle elasticity. They also aid in the prevention of injuries by gradually increasing your heart rate and warming up your joints. Seniors over 60 can safely and effectively begin their fitness program with these easy workouts.

Why Warm-up Exercises are effective

1. Improved Blood Flow: Warm-up activities improve blood flow all over your body. This helps your muscles get the oxygen and nutrition they need for the next session.

2. Increased Flexibility: Warm-up activities increase your range of motion and flexibility by having you execute light rotations and stretches. This can enhance general mobility and lessen the chance of strained muscles.

3. Joint Lubrication: Synovial fluid production is stimulated by warm-up exercises, and this fluid lubricates the joints. This lessens resistance and makes workout action more smoother.

4. Mental Preparation: Engaging in warm-up exercises helps shift your focus to the present moment, allowing you to mentally prepare for the workout ahead. It can also help improve concentration and coordination.

Safety Tips

---

1. Start Slowly: As your body warms up, start with slower motions and progressively build the intensity. Pay attention to your body and refrain from overexerting yourself.

2. Maintain Correct Form: Throughout the warm-up exercises, be mindful of your posture. Avoid slouching, sit up straight in your chair, and adjust your spine.

3. Remain Hydrated: To stay hydrated, don't forget to sip water before, during, and after your warm-up exercises.

4. Adjust as Needed: If a certain movement hurts or is uncomfortable, adjust or skip that exercise. It's critical to operate inside your own comfort zone and skill set.

5. Speak with Your Doctor: Before beginning any fitness program, speak with your healthcare practitioner if you have any underlying medical ailments or concerns.

1. Neck stretches and rotations

---

1. Take a tall seat in your chair with your feet flat on the ground.

2. Bring your right ear close to your right shoulder as you gently tilt your head to the right. Hold on for a few seconds.

3. Repeat on the left side after coming back to the center.

4. After then, carefully turn your head in a circular motion, moving your chin to your chest, then to the right, left and back. Carry out the opposite direction.

2. Shoulder rolls and shrugs

1. Relax your arms and let them hang by your sides.

2. Roll your shoulders forward in a circular pattern, increasing the size of the circles as you go. Repeat for 10-15 seconds.

3. Change course and roll your shoulders backward for another 10-15 seconds.

4. Raise your shoulders to your ears, hold there for a brief period of time, then release. Repeat 8-10 times.

3. Wrist and ankle circles

1.   Extend your arms forward, palms facing down.

2.   Gently rotate your wrists in a clockwise and counterclockwise direction. Repeat for 10-15 seconds.

3.   Point your toes forward and lift your heels off the ground.

4.   Make a clockwise and counterclockwise circle with your ankles. Repeat for 10-15 seconds.

4. Marching in place

---

1. With your feet flat on the ground, sit up straight in your chair.

2. Raise your right knee to your chest and then return it to its original position.

3. Repeat on your left knee, switching back and forth between the two.

4. Continue marching in place for 30 seconds to 1 minute, gradually increasing the pace.

5. Seated torso twists

1. With your feet flat on the ground, sit up straight in your chair.

2. For support, place your hands on your thighs or grip the chair's sides.

3. Maintaining your hips and lower body pointing forward, slowly twist your upper body to the right.

4. After a few seconds of holding the stretch, turn back to the center.

5. Move to the left side and repeat the motion.

6. Perform 8–10 reputations on each side, alternating between right and left twists.

6. Ankle pumps

1. With your feet flat on the ground, sit up straight in your chair.

2. While maintaining your heels on the ground, raise your toes toward the ceiling.

3. Reposition your toes lower.

4. Next, press your heels down towards the floor, lifting your toes up.

5. Do 10–12 repetitions of the ankle pumps, switching between lifting your heels and raising your toes.

7. Arm Circles

---

1. Arrange your arms out to the sides while sitting tall and keeping your feet flat on the ground.

2. Make small circles with your arms, gradually increasing the size of the circles.

3. change course and make circles in the other direction.

4. Perform 8-10 repetitions in each direction.

8. Seated Toe Touches

---

1. Take a tall sit with your feet flat on the ground, legs extended in front of you.

2. Reach your arms forward and slowly bend forward at the waist, reaching towards your toes.

3. When you feel a slight stretch in your hamstrings, stop for a moment.

4. Return to the starting position and repeat for 8-10 repetitions.

9. Shoulder Blade Squeezes

1. **Maintain a straight posture while sitting tall and keeping your arms at your sides.**

2. **Pull your shoulder blades toward your spine by squeezing them together.**

3. **Squeeze for a brief period of time, then release.**

4. **Make 10–12 repetitions, paying particular attention to engaging your upper back muscles.**

10. Seated Side Leg Raises

1. Sit tall with your feet flat on the ground.

2. Keeping your leg straight, raise one out to the side.

3. After a brief period of time at the highest height, lower your leg back down.

4. Continue with the opposite leg.

5. Perform 8-10 repetitions on each leg, engaging your hip muscles.

It's important to include warm-up activities in your routine to get your body prepared for the chair exercises ahead. These activities enhance blood flow, improve flexibility and also help you mentally prepare for the workout. Always put safety first by taking it slow, using the right form, and seeing a doctor when necessary. Spending some time warming up prepares you for a secure and productive workout. Now that you're ready, let's examine the upper body workouts for seniors over 60 in the following chapter.

Chapter 2

Upper body exercises

Greetings and welcome to Chapter 2 of our senior over-60 chair workouts. We'll concentrate on exercises that are meant to tone and strengthen your upper body. Sustaining upper body strength is crucial for performing daily tasks like reaching, lifting, and carrying things. These are accessible and convenient exercises that you can perform from the comfort of your chair. You'll maintain your independence, strengthen your posture, and improve your strength by adding these upper body exercises to your routine.

Why Upper Body Exercises are effective

1. Enhanced Strength: Strengthening your arms, shoulders, chest, and back muscles can be achieved with regular upper body exercises. This can lessen your chance of developing muscular imbalances or weakness and enhance your capacity to carry out daily tasks.

2. Improved Bone Health: Resistance training can help increase bone density and reduce the risk of osteoporosis. Examples of these exercises include chair push-ups and seated rowing motions with resistance bands.

3. Posture Improvement: By building stronger upper body muscles, you can improve your posture and lessen the strain on your back and neck.

4. Functional Independence: Being able to carry out tasks like lifting groceries, opening doors, and carrying objects with ease is made possible by having a strong upper body.

Safety Tips

---

1. Employ Correct Form: Throughout each exercise, be mindful of your posture and technique. Keep your back straight, contract your abs, and refrain from jerking or straining.

2. Start with Light Resistance: If you're going to use weights, start with smaller ones or use resistance bands or water bottles instead. As your strength increases, gradually increase the resistance.

3. Take Breaks When Needed: Pay attention to your body's needs and take breaks if you start to feel tired or uncomfortable. It's crucial to go at your own pace and build up to more intensity gradually.

4. Refrain from Overexertion: Although pushing yourself to the limit is vital, refrain from going overboard. If you feel any sharp pain or dizziness, stop right away.

5. Remain Hydrated: To stay hydrated, don't forget to sip water before, during, and after your workout.

1. Seated arm raises

---

1. Take a tall seat in your chair, keeping your arms at your sides and your feet flat on the ground.

2. Slowly lift both arms forward, and keep them straight until they are parallel to the floor.

3. After maintaining the posture for a little while, drop your arms once more.

4. Perform 10-12 repetitions.

2. Push-ups with a chair

1. Grip the seat with your hands placed shoulder-width apart on the chair's edge.

2. Step forward with your feet so that your body forms a diagonal line and your back is straight.

3. Bend your elbows and lower your body toward the chair, keeping your elbows close to your sides.

4. Return to the starting position by pushing back up.

5. Complete 8–10 repetitions, varying the difficulty by moving your feet in front of or behind the chair.

3. Seated rowing motion with resistance bands

---

1. Loop a resistance band around your feet while sitting up straight and keeping your feet flat on the ground.

2. Hold the ends of the resistance band with your palms facing each other.

3. Pull the band in the direction of your chest while bringing your shoulder blades together.

4. Release slowly and perform 10–12 repetitions.

4. Seated tricep dips

1. Place your hands on the chair's edge with your fingers pointing forward.

2. Slide your bottom off the chair, supporting your weight with your hands.

3. Keeping your back close to the chair, bend your elbows and lower your body toward the floor.

4. Return to the starting position by pushing back up.

5. Complete 8–10 repetitions, varying the difficulty by moving your feet in front of or behind the chair.

5. Seated shoulder press

1. Hold a pair of dumbbells or water bottles in your hands while sitting tall and keeping your feet flat on the ground.

2. Start with placing your hands shoulder-level with the palms facing forward.

3. Lift the weights above your head while fully extending your arms.

4. Reducing the weights gradually back down to shoulder level.

5. Complete 8–10 repetitions, varying the weight according to your capacity.

6. Seated bicep curls

1. Hold a pair of dumbbells or a water bottle in your hands, palms facing forward, while sitting tall and keeping your feet flat on the ground.

2. Curl the weights slowly in the direction of your shoulders while maintaining your elbows close to your sides.

3. Squeeze your biceps as you pause at the top, then slowly lower the weights back down.

4. Perform 8-10 repetitions, varying the weight as necessary.

7. Seated Chest Press

---

1. Maintain a straight posture while sitting tall and hold a pair of dumbbells or water bottles at chest level.

2. Extend your arms fully without locking your elbows as you push the weights forward.

3. Return the weights to your chest gradually.

4. Complete 8–10 repetitions, varying the weight to suit your comfort zone.

8. Seated Reverse Fly

1. Hold a pair of dumbbells or water bottles in your hands while sitting tall and keeping your feet flat on the ground.

2. With your palms facing each other, extend your arms in front of you.

3. Squeeze your shoulder blades together while extending your arms to the sides.

4. Go back to the beginning position slowly.

5. Make 8–10 repetitions, paying particular attention to using your upper back muscles.

9. Seated Overhead Tricep Extension

1. Hold a dumbbell or water bottle with both hands and raise it overhead while sitting tall and keeping your feet flat on the ground.

2. Lower the weight behind your head by bending your elbows.

3. Extend your arms, lifting the weight back overhead.

4. Perform 8-10 repetitions, varying the weight as necessary.

10. Seated Arm Circles with Resistance Bands

---

1. Sit tall with your feet flat on the ground and place a resistance band around your wrists.

2. With your palms facing down, extend your arms out to the sides.

3. Using your arms, make tiny circles, progressively increasing the size of the circles.

4. After 10-15 seconds, reverse the direction and make circles in the opposite direction.

5. Perform 8-10 times in each direction.

Strengthening your upper body through these exercises will help you become more independent overall and with better posture. Always remember to put safety first by using appropriate form, easing up on the resistance at first, and paying attention to your body's cues. You'll reap the rewards of a stronger upper body with perseverance and steady advancement. We'll look at strengthening and stabilizing exercises for your lower body in the upcoming chapter.

Chapter 3

---

exercises for the lower body

Greetings and welcome to Chapter 3 of our senior over-60 chair workouts. We'll concentrate on exercises that target the muscles in your lower body. Strengthening your legs, hips, and buttocks is crucial for maintaining balance, stability, and mobility, which are essential for performing daily activities and maintaining an active and independent lifestyle. These chair workouts are made to be simple, accessible, and efficient at increasing the strength and flexibility of your lower body.

Why Lower Body Exercises are effective

1. Enhanced Leg Strength: Consistent lower body workouts help strengthen your leg muscles, such as your calves, hamstrings, and quadriceps. This can make it easier for you to walk, climb stairs, and carry out other weight-bearing tasks.

2. Improved Balance and Stability: Building muscle in your hip and buttock area can help you feel more balanced and stable overall, which lowers your chance of accidents and falls.

3. Joint Flexibility: Exercises for the lower body help preserve or enhance the range of motion and decrease stiffness in your hip, knee, and ankle joints.

4. Functional Independence: Being able to independently navigate different types of terrain, carry out household chores, and participate in recreational activities is made possible by having strong lower body muscles.

Safety Tips

---

1. Chair Stability: To avoid any mishaps or slips during the exercises, make sure your chair is stable and placed on a non-slip surface.

2. Correct Form: Keep your posture straight during the workouts. Keep your shoulders from rounding, sit tall, and contract your core muscles.

3. Gradual Progression: As you develop strength and flexibility, begin with exercises that feel comfortable for you and progressively up the number of repetitions, the intensity, or the range of motion.

4. Listen to Your Body: During the exercises, be aware of any pain or discomfort. Stop the exercise and see a medical professional if you feel any severe or persistent pain.

5. Stay Hydrated: To stay hydrated and preserve optimal physical function, drink water before, during, and after your workout.

1. Seated leg lifts

---

1. With your feet flat on the ground, sit up straight in your chair.

2. With your knee slightly bent, extend one leg straight out in front of you.

3. Raise your extended leg as high as comfortable, then lower it back down.

4. Repeat for 10-12 repetitions on each leg.

2. Chair squats

---

1. Place your feet shoulder-width apart in front of your chair.

2. Maintain your weight in your heels as you slowly lower your body toward the chair as if you were going to sit down.

3. Without completely sitting down, hover just above the chair and then stand back up.

4. Complete 8–10 repetitions, varying the squat depth according to your comfort and strength.

3. Seated heel-to-toe raises

---

1. Take a tall sit with your feet flat on the ground.

2. Raising yourself onto your toes, lift your heels off the ground.

3. Return your heels back to the ground.

4. Repeat for 10-12 repetitions, emphasizing balance and control.

4. Seated knee extensions

1. With your feet flat on the ground, sit up straight in your chair.

2. Stretch one leg out in front of you, attempting to keep your knee as straight as you can.

3. After maintaining the extended posture for a little while, bend your knee and place your foot back on the ground.

4. Repeat for 10-12 repetitions on each leg, switching between them.

5. Seated marching

1. Sit tall with your feet flat on the ground.

2. Raise one foot off the ground and bring your knee closer to your chest.

3. Return your foot to the floor, then do the same with the other leg.

4. For 30 to 60 seconds, keep switching between your legs as if you were marching in place.

6. Seated side leg raises

1. Sit tall with your feet flat on the ground.

2. While keeping your knee straight, raise one leg out to the side.

3. After a brief period of time, return your leg to its lower position.

4. Repeat for 10-12 repetitions on each leg, switching between them.

7. Seated Calf Raises

---

1. Sit tall with your feet flat on the ground.

2. Lift your heels off the ground, rising up onto your toes.

3. Return your heels to the ground.

4. Concentrate on maintaining control and using your calf muscles as you perform 10–12 repetitions.

8. Seated Inner Thigh Squeezes

1. Take a tall seat with your legs slightly apart, knees bent, and feet flat on the ground.

2. Put a tiny pillow or exercise ball in between your knees.

3. Squeeze your knees together to activate the muscles in your inner thighs.

4. Hold the squeeze for a short while, then release.

5. Repeat for 10-12 repetitions, focusing on control and maintaining proper posture.

9. Seated Glute Bridges

---

1. With your knees bent and your feet flat on the ground, take a seat at the edge of your chair.

2. For support, rest your hands on the chair's sides.

3. Squeeze your glutes as you raise your hips off the chair.

4. After a brief period of time, return your hips to their lower position.

5. Perform 8-10 repetitions, paying particular attention to using your glute muscles.

10. Seated Ankle Circles

1. Take a tall sit with your feet flat on the ground.

2. Raising one foot off the ground, turn your ankle clockwise in a circular motion.

3. After 10-15 seconds, change course and rotate counterclockwise in circles.

4. With the other foot, repeat the ankle circles.

5. Perform 8-10 repetitions in each direction.

You can greatly increase the strength, balance, and general mobility of your lower body by including these exercises into your routine. Always put safety first by following appropriate form, making small progress, and paying attention to your body's cues. You'll reap the rewards of a stronger and more flexible lower body with perseverance and dedication. We'll look at some exercises in the upcoming chapter that will help you become more flexible overall and relax.

Chapter 4

Core exercises

Greetings and welcome to Chapter 4 of our senior over-60 chair workouts. We'll concentrate on exercises that work your core muscles in this chapter. Sustaining stability, balance, and good posture requires a strong core. Your back, side, and abdominal muscles will all get stronger with the aid of these chair exercises, which will support a strong and functional core. You can increase your general strength, stability, and flexibility by including these exercises in your routine, which will help you continue to be active and independent.

Why Core Exercises are effective

1. Better Posture: By strengthening the muscles that support your spine, core exercises help you keep better posture all day. This can enhance general body alignment and relieve back pain.

2. Improved Stability and Balance: You can move with more stability and less risk of falls and injuries when you have a strong core.

3. Enhanced Functional Strength: Bending, lifting, and twisting are just a few of the everyday tasks that require the use of core muscles. These movements may become more effortless and effective with the strengthening of these muscles.

4. Improved Spine Health: By increasing spinal flexibility, lowering the risk of disc degeneration, and easing the strain on the back muscles, core exercises help to improve the health of your spine.

Safety Tips

---

1. Appropriate Body Alignment: Keep your posture correct during the exercises. Avoid slumping or overarching your back, sit up straight, and contract your core muscles.

2. Gradual Progression: As your core strength increases, start with exercises that feel comfortable for you and progressively up the number of repetitions or intensity.

3. Breathing and Control: Pay attention to how you naturally breathe and how you keep your composure during each exercise. Refrain from using jerky movements or holding your breath.

4. Adjust as Needed: Adjust or omit a specific exercise if it hurts or is uncomfortable. Work within your comfort zone and pay attention to your body.

5. Warm-Up and Cool-Down: Start every workout with a light warm-up, like shoulder rolls or a march in place. Finish with a cool-down and some light stretches to help you become more flexible and calm.

1. Seated trunk twists

1. Take a tall seat in your chair, placing your hands on your thighs and your feet flat on the ground.

2. With your hips pointing forward, slowly turn your torso to one side.

3. Hold the twist for a little while, then return to the center.

4. Repeat on the other side.

5. Complete 8-10 repetitions on each side, making sure your movements are deliberate.

2. Abdominal contractions while seated

1. Sit tall with your feet flat on the floor and hands resting on your thighs.

2. Inhale deeply, then contract your abdominal muscles by drawing your belly button toward your spine as you exhale.

3. After a few seconds of holding the contraction, release it.

4. Repeat for 10-12 repetitions, paying close attention to how your core muscles are being used.

3. Seated side bends

1. Sit tall with your feet flat on the ground and arms relaxed by your sides.

2. Raise one arm overhead while bending slightly to the other side.

3. Return to the center and repeat on the other side.

4. Focus on the stretch and contraction of your side muscles as you complete 8–10 repetitions on each side.

4. Seated pelvic tilts

1. With your feet flat on the ground, sit up straight in your chair.

2. Place your hands on your hips or thighs.

3. Tilt your pelvis forward gradually while slightly arching your lower back.

4. Next, round your lower back by tilting your pelvis backward.

5. Continue rocking in this manner, being mindful to use your core muscles.

6. Perform 8-10 repetitions while keeping your movements under control.

5. Seated knee-to-chest lifts

---

1. With your feet flat on the ground, sit up straight in your chair.

2. Bring one knee up to your chest and give it a gentle hand hug.

3. Feel the stretch in your hips and lower back as you hold this position for a short while.

4. Release and repeat with the other leg.

5. Alternate between legs for 8-10 repetitions per side.

6. Seated Russian twists

1. Take a tall seat with your knees bent and your feet flat on the ground.

2. Lean back slightly while maintaining good posture.

3. Clasp your hands in front of your chest.

4. Turn your torso to one side and move your clasped hands in that direction.

5. Go back to the center and carry out the opposite side.

6. Complete 8–10 repetitions on each side, concentrating on deliberate twisting motions.

7. Seated Spine Rotation

---

1. Maintain a tall seat by placing your hands on your thighs and your feet flat on the ground.

2. Twist from your waist to one side while slowly rotating your upper body.

3. For a brief moment, hold the twist while feeling how your back and abdominal muscles stretch and contract.

4. Go back to the center and do the opposite side.

5. Complete 8–10 repetitions on each side, making sure your movements are deliberate.

8. Seated Leg Extensions with Rotation

1. Take a tall sit with your feet flat on the ground.

2. With your knee slightly bent, extend one leg in front of you.

3. Turn your torso in the direction of the extended leg as you extend it.

4. Go back to the center and carry out the opposite side.

5. Work your leg and core muscles during 8–10 repetitions on each side.

9. Seated Bicycle Crunches

---

1. Maintain a straight posture while sitting tall and place your hands behind your head.

2. Raise one knee to your chest and twist your torso so that your elbow on the other side of the knee comes in contact with the knee.

3. Return to the starting position and repeat with the other knee and elbow.

4. Perform 8–10 repetitions on each side, alternating between the sides.

10. Seated Plank Hold

---

1. Take a seat at the edge of the chair with your hands shoulder-width apart on the seat.

2. With your hands supporting you, walk your feet backward until your body forms a straight line from your head to your heels.

3. Using your core muscles, hold the position for 10-20 seconds, being mindful of your alignment.

4. As your core strength increases, gradually extend the duration of the plank hold.

You can improve your posture, stability, and general functional strength by including these core exercises in your routine. They will also help you develop a strong and stable core. Always keep safety first by using appropriate form, increasing gradually, and paying attention to your body's cues. You'll reap the rewards of a more robust and resilient core with perseverance and consistency. We will examine exercises that encourage flexibility and relaxation in the upcoming chapter.

Chapter 5

Stretching exercises

Greetings and welcome to Chapter 6 of our senior over-60 chair workouts. This chapter will concentrate on stretches that will increase joint mobility and encourage flexibility. Stretching is an essential component of any exercise routine, as it helps to lengthen and loosen tight muscles, enhance range of motion, and alleviate muscle stiffness. Stretching while seated can help you stay flexible and keep your body supple and agile. These exercises are safe, easy to use, and effective.

Why Stretching Exercises are effective

1. Greater Flexibility: Stretching on a regular basis can help you become more flexible in your muscles and joints, which can enhance your general mobility and make daily tasks easier.

2. Improved Joint Health: Stretching exercises encourage the flow of synovial fluid, which lubricates and nourishes the joints while easing pain and stiffness.

3. Better Posture: Stretching relieves tension and lengthens tense muscles, which helps you maintain better alignment and posture.

4. Stress Relief: Stretching exercises can help to promote relaxation and reduce stress by having a calming effect on the body and mind.

Safety Tips

1. Warm-Up: It's crucial to warm up your muscles with mild movements like shoulder rolls or place-to-place marches before beginning any stretching exercises. In addition to improving blood flow, this gets your muscles ready for stretching.

2. Mild and Gradual: Pain should never be experienced when stretching. Aim for comfortable, gentle stretches; steer clear of jerky or bouncing motions. Over time, progressively increase the length and intensity of your stretches.

3. Breathe and Relax: Don't forget to take deep breaths and unwind during each stretch. Breathe out as the stretch gets deeper; do not hold your breath.

4. Individual Comfort: Since everyone has a different degree of flexibility, you should only stretch until you feel a slight tug or strain in your muscles. Never push yourself past your comfort zone when stretching.

5. Balance and Stability: Before beginning the exercises, make sure your chair is secure and stable. If additional stability is required, position the chair against a wall or use one with armrests.

1. Seated hamstring stretch

1. With one leg extended straight out in front of you, take a seat close to the edge of your chair.

2. Maintain a straight back while bending forward from the hips and reaching for your toes.

3. Feeling a light stretch in the back of your thigh as you hold the stretch for 20 to 30 seconds.

4. Change legs and perform the stretch again on the opposite side.

5. Stretch each leg for 2-3 repetitions, progressively going deeper if it feels comfortable.

2. Seated calf stretches

---

1. Take a tall sit with your feet flat on the ground.

2. With your toes pointing upward and your heel on the ground, extend one leg out in front of you.

3. Feel the stretch in your calf as you gently bring your toes closer to your body.

4. Release the stretch after 20 to 30 seconds of holding it.

5. Stretch the other leg once more.

6. Perform 2-3 repetitions on each leg, focusing on relaxing into the stretch.

3. Seated chest and shoulder stretches

1. Maintain a tall seat by placing your hands on your thighs and your feet flat on the ground.

2. Squeeze your shoulder blades together by interlacing your fingers behind your back.

3. Feel a stretch across your shoulders and chest as you gently raise your hands upward.

4. Release the stretch after 20 to 30 seconds of holding it.

5. Complete 2-3 repetitions, paying close attention to your posture throughout the stretch.

4. Seated spinal twist

1. Maintain a tall posture by placing your hands on your thighs and your feet flat on the ground.

2. Turn your body to one side and steady yourself by resting your other hand on the outside of your thigh.

3. Looking over your shoulder, slowly rotate your upper body.

4. Hold the stretch for 20 to 30 seconds, allowing your spine to gently twist during that time.

5. Go back to the center and carry out the opposite side.

6. Perform 2-3 repetitions on each side, making sure to keep your twist comfortable.

5. Seated hip stretch

1. Take a seat close to the edge of the chair so that one ankle rests on the knee of the other.

2. Feel the stretch in your hip as you gently press down on the raised knee while maintaining a straight back.

3. Release the stretch after 20 to 30 seconds of holding it.

4. Change legs and perform the stretch again on the opposite side.

5. Perform 2-3 repetitions on each side, gradually deepening the stretch if comfortable.

6. Seated shoulder and neck stretch

1. Take a tall sit, keeping your arms at your sides and your feet flat on the ground.

2. Extend one arm across your chest, supporting it with the other hand on your upper arm.

3. Feel the back of your neck and shoulder stretches as you slowly bring your arm up to your chest.

4. Release the stretch after 20 to 30 seconds of holding it.

5. Extend the other arm in the same manner.

6. Perform 2-3 repetitions on each side, focusing on relaxing into the stretch.

7. Seated Upper Back Stretch

1. Maintain a tall posture by placing your hands on your thighs and your feet flat on the ground.

2. With your palms pointing outward, interlace your fingers in front of you.

3. Extend your upper back, feeling a stretch between your shoulder blades as you push your hands away from your body.

4. Release the stretch after 20 to 30 seconds of holding it.

5. Perform 2-3 repetitions, paying close attention to your posture the entire time.

8. Seated Quadriceps Stretch

---

1. Sit tall with your feet flat on the ground.

2. Place your heel on the ground and extend one leg straight out in front of you.

3. Bend the other knee slightly and place your hand over your ankle or lower leg.

4. Pull your heel towards your buttocks, feeling a stretch in the front of your thigh.

5. Release the stretch after 20 to 30 seconds of holding it.

6. Stretch the other leg once more.

7. On each leg, Perform 2-3 repetitions concentrating on relaxing into the stretch.

9. Seated Neck Side Stretch

---

1. Take a tall Sit with your feet flat on the ground and arms relaxed by your sides.

2. Tilt your head so that your ear is closer to your shoulder.

3. Feel the stretch in your neck as you gently press your hand against the other side of your head.

4. Release the stretch after 20 to 30 seconds of holding it.

5. Stretch the opposite side again.

6. Perform 2-3 repetitions on each side, being mindful to keep the stretch comfortable.

10. Seated Ankle Circles

---

1. Take a tall Sit with your feet flat on the ground.

2. Elevate your foot off the ground and start circling your ankle in a clockwise manner.

3. Perform 10-15 circles, then turn the motion counterclockwise.

4. Use the other foot to complete the exercise again.

5. Perform 2-3 sets on each foot, focusing on smooth and controlled movements.

You can increase your general well-being, joint mobility, and flexibility by including these stretching exercises in your routine. Always put safety first by warming up, doing light stretches, and paying attention to your body's limitations. Stretching on a regular basis will help you keep your body flexible and agile, which will keep you independent and active. We will look at relaxation techniques in the upcoming chapter to help you feel at ease and less stressed.

Conclusion

You've made great progress in maintaining your independence, staying active, and building your strength and flexibility by adding these simple and accessible workouts into your daily routine.

I have presented several chapters in this book, each of which focuses on a distinct body part and includes targeted workouts to work that particular area. Based on your preference and fitness objectives, you may now choose from a wide range of alternatives, including warm-up exercises, upper body, lower body, core, and stretching routines.

It's impossible to overestimate the advantages of regular exercise for seniors. You have raised your quality of life in general and your physical health in particular by performing chair exercises. Frequent exercise helps strengthen muscles, promote mood and mental health, improve balance and coordination, and strengthen the heart.

Always keep in mind that your safety comes first when doing any kind of workout. Before beginning a new fitness routine, always listen to your body and see your doctor, especially if you have any underlying medical concerns.

It's also crucial to begin softly and increase the duration and intensity of your workouts gradually. In order to avoid injuries, make sure you follow the directions for each exercise carefully and ask for help if necessary.

Maintaining consistency is essential. To reap the greatest rewards, try to include these chair exercises into your monthly or daily schedule. Your general health and well-being can be significantly improved by even brief exercise sessions.

Finally, remember to have fun during the process. Make activities that you truly enjoy a part of your routine so that exercising can be a source of joy and fulfillment. Choose an activity that makes you happy and keep moving, it might be yoga, resistance band training, or dancing to your favorite music!

I appreciate you for embarking on this path to put your health and wellbeing first. You are encouraging people to live healthier lives by being independent and active, and you are also providing a good example for those around you. Keep up the good effort and I hope you have a long, fulfilling life filled with activity and vibrancy.

Thank you for choosing "Chair Exercises for Seniors over 60" as your guide to staying active, independent, and boosting your strength and flexibility. I hope you have found this book informative and helpful in your fitness journey.

I would greatly appreciate it if you could take a moment to rate and review this book. Your feedback is valuable to me as it helps me improve and provide better content in the future. Your positive review will also encourage others to discover the benefits of chair exercises and lead a healthier lifestyle.

Your honest opinion is highly appreciated, and I thank you in advance for your support.

Stay active, stay independent, and keep moving!